Soups Collection for Plant-Based Diet

Quick and Tasty Soups Recipes to Start Your Plant-Based Diet and Boost Your Metabolism

Dave Ingram

Table of contents

Coconut Watercress Soup

Preparation Time: 10 minutes

Cooking Time: 20 minutes

Servings: 4

Ingredients:

1 teaspoon coconut oil 1 onion, diced

¾ cup coconut milk

Directions:

1.   Add the onion to the melted coconut oil and cook until soft, about 5 minutes, then add the peas and the water. Add the watercress, mint, salt, and pepper.

2.   Cover and simmer for 5 minutes. Stir in the coconut milk, and purée the soup until smooth in a blender or with an immersion blender.

3.   Try this soup with any other fresh, leafy green— anything from spinach to collard greens to arugula to swiss chard.

Nutrition:

Calories: 160 Fat: 5g Carbs: 25g Proteins: 2g

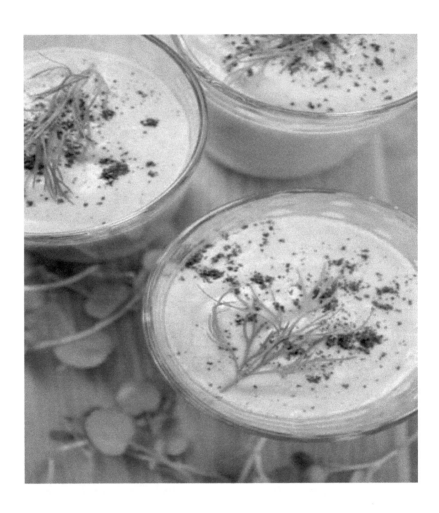

Roasted Red Pepper and Butternut Squash Soup

Preparation Time: 10 minutes

Cooking Time: 45 minutes

Servings: 6

Ingredients:

1 small butternut squash 1 tablespoon olive oil

1 teaspoon sea salt 2 red bell peppers 1 yellow onion

1 head garlic

2 cups water, or vegetable broth Zest and juice of 1 lime

1 to 2 tablespoons tahini Pinch cayenne pepper

½ teaspoon ground coriander

½ teaspoon ground cumin Toasted squash seeds (optional)

Directions:

1.   Preheat the oven to 350°F.

2.   Prepare the squash for roasting by cutting it in half lengthwise and scooping out the seeds. Reserve the seeds if desired.

3.   Put the halves skin-side down in a large baking dish. Put it in the oven while you prepare the rest of the vegetables.

4.   Prepare the peppers the same way, except they do not need to be poked.

5.   Slice the onion in half and rub oil on the exposed faces.

6.   Add peppers, onion, and garlic, and roast for another 20 minutes. Optionally, you can toast the squash seeds by putting them in the oven in a separate baking dish 10 to 15 minutes before the vegetables are finished.

7.   Keep a close eye on them.

8.   Scoop into a blender.

9.   Chop the pepper roughly, remove the onion skin and chop the onion roughly, and squeeze the garlic cloves out of the head, all into the pot or blender. Add the water, the lime zest and juice, and the tahini. Purée the soup, adding more water if you like, to your desired consistency. Season with salt, cayenne, coriander, and

cumin. Serve garnished with toasted squash seeds (if using).

Nutrition:

Calories: 156 Protein: 4g Fat: 11g Carbs: 22g

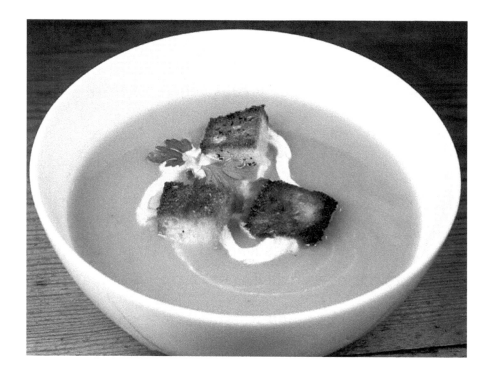

Cauliflower Spinach Soup

Preparation Time: 30 minutes

Cooking Time: 25 minutes

Servings: 5

Ingredients:

1/2 cup unsweetened coconut milk 5 oz. fresh spinach, chopped

5 watercress, chopped 8 cups vegetable stock

1 lb cauliflower, chopped Salt

Directions:

1.   Add stock and cauliflower in a large saucepan and bring to boil over medium heat for 15 minutes.

2.   Add spinach and watercress and cook for another 10 minutes.

3.   Pureè until smooth.

4.   Add coconut milk and stir well. Season with salt.

5.   Stir well and serve hot.

Nutrition:

Calories: 271 Fat: 3.7g Carbs: 54g Proteins: 6.5g

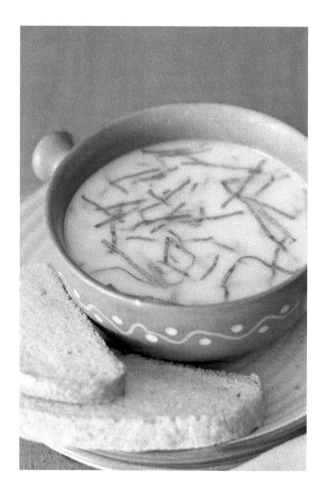

Avocado Mint Soup

Preparation Time: 10 minutes

Cooking Time: 10 minutes

Servings: 2

Ingredients:

2 avocado 1 cup coconut milk

2 romaine lettuce leaves 20 fresh mint leaves

1 tbsp lime juice 1/6 tsp salt

Directions:

1.   Add all ingredients into the blender and blend until smooth. The soup should be thick, not as a puree.

2.   Pour into the serving bowls and place them in the refrigerator for 10 minutes.

3.   Stir well and serve chilled.

Nutrition:

Calories: 377 Fat: 14.9g Carbs: 20.7g Protein: 6.4g

Creamy Squash Soup

Preparation Time: 10 minutes

Cooking Time: 25 minutes

Servings: 8

Ingredients:

3 cups butternut squash, chopped

1 ½ cups unsweetened coconut milk 1 tbsp coconut oil

1 tsp dried onion flakes

 1 tbsp curry powder 4 cups water

1 garlic clove

1 tsp kosher salt

Directions:

1.   Add squash, coconut oil, onion flakes, curry powder, water, garlic, and salt into a large saucepan. Bring to boil over high heat.

2.   Simmer for 25 minutes.

3.   Puree the soup using a blender. Mix with the coconut milk, then cook for 4 minutes.

4.   Stir well and serve hot.

Nutrition:

Calories: 271 Fat: 3.7g Carbs: 54g Protein:6.5g

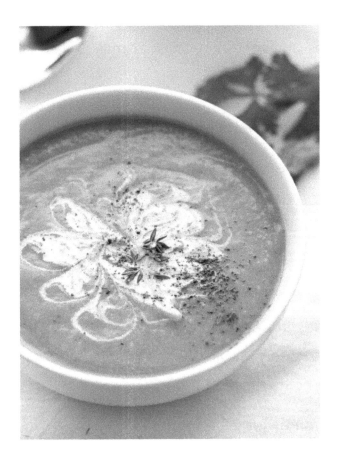

Zucchini Soup

Preparation Time: 10 minutes

Cooking Time: 15 minutes

Servings: 8

Ingredients:

2   ½ lbs zucchini, peeled and sliced 1/3 cup basil leaves

4 cups vegetable stock 4 garlic cloves, chopped 2 tbsp olive oil

1 medium onion, diced Pepper

Salt

Directions:

1.   Heat the extra-virgin olive oil.

2.   Add zucchini and onion and sauté until softened. Add garlic and sauté for a minute.

3.   Put the vegetable stock and simmer for 15 minutes.

4.   Remove from heat. Stir in basil and puree the soup using a blender until smooth and creamy. Season with pepper and salt.

5.   Stir well and serve.

Nutrition:

Calories: 434 Fat: 35g Carbs: 27g Protein: 6.7g

Can Chili

Preparation time: 5 minutes

Cook time: 30 minutes

Serves 6

Ingredients:

1 (28-ounce / 794-g) can crushed tomatoes

1 (15-ounce /425-g) can low-sodium black beans

1 (15-ounce /425-g) can low-sodium cannellini beans 1 (15-ounce /425-g) can low-sodium chickpeas

1 tbsp chili 1 tsp garlic 1 tsp onion

½ teaspoon ground cumin

½ teaspoon red pepper flakes (optional)

Directions:

1.   In a large stockpot, combine the tomatoes, black beans, cannellini beans, chickpeas, liquids with chili powder, garlic powder, onion powder, cumin, and red

pepper flakes (if using). Bring the chili to a boil over medium-high heat.

2.   Let it simmer for 25 minutes, and serve.

Nutrition Per Serving:

calories: 185 | fat: 1g | carbs: 33g | protein: 11g | fiber: 13g

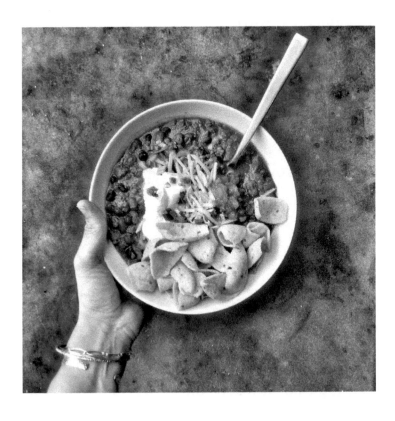

Three Bean Chili

Preparation time: 25 minutes

Cook time: 2 hours 10 minutes

Serves 12

Ingredients:

1 cup black beans 1 cup pinto beans 1 cup kidney beans

6½ cups water, divided

1 red bell pepper

1 green bell pepper 1 cup celery

1 cup chopped onion

3 cloves garlic, minced

½ tablespoon ground cumin

¼ cup chili powder

¼ tsp red pepper flakes 1 tsp oregano

1 (4-ounce/ 113-g) can chopped green chilies

1 (28-ounce / 794-g) can crushed tomatoes

Directions:

1.   Add the beans and 6 cups of water to a large pot over medium heat and bring to a boil. Allow to boil for 2 minutes and remove from the heat. Cover the pot and let sit for 1 hour.

2.   Combine the bell pepper, celery, onion, garlic, and remaining ½ cup of water in another pot. Sauté for about 6 minutes, or until the vegetables are tender.

3.   Stir in the beans and their water, cumin, chili powder, red pepper, and oregano, and let it boil. Simmer covered for 1 hour, stirring occasionally.

4.   Add the chilies and tomatoes and stir well. Cook for an additional 1 hour, stirring occasionally.

5.   Allow cooling for 5 minutes before ladling into bowls to serve.

Nutrition Per Serving:

calories: 177 | fat: 2g | carbs: 29g | protein: 9g | fiber: 9g

Basic Vegetable Stock

Preparation time: 15 minutes

Cook time: 45 minutes

Makes 2 quarts

Ingredients:

2 large leeks, chopped and rinsed

2 stalks celery, including some leaves, coarsely chopped
2 large carrots, peeled and coarsely chopped

1 bunch green onions, chopped

4 cloves garlic 6 sprigs parsley 4 sprigs fresh thyme

2 bay leaves

10 cups water

Directions:

1.   Bring the ingredients to a boil. Let it simmer for 45 minutes. Let it cool before serving. Refrigerate for up to seven days.

Succotash Soup with Basil

Preparation time: 10 minutes

Cook time: 35 minutes

Serves 4 to 6

Ingredients:

4 leeks 1 large red bell pepper, diced into ½-inch cubes

4 cloves garlic 3 teaspoons thyme 6 cups vegetable stock

1 (10-ounce / 283-g) package frozen edamame, shelled

4 cups fresh corn or 2 (10-ounce / 283-g) packages frozen corn

½ cup chopped fresh basil

Sea salt and black pepper, to taste

Directions:

1.   Heat a large pot over medium heat. Add the leeks and red bell pepper and cook for 7 to 8 minutes, until the leeks start to brown. Add the garlic and thyme and sauté for 1 minute. Add the vegetable stock, edamame, and

corn, and bring to a boil. Leti t simmer for 20 to 25 minutes. Add the chopped basil and cook for another minute.

2.   Remove the soup from heat and season to taste with salt and pepper.

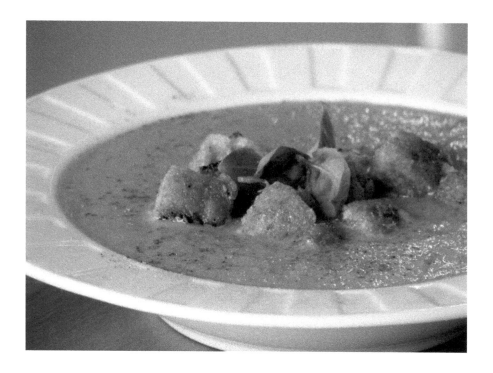

Black Bean and Sweet Potato Stew

Preparation time: 15 minutes

Cook time: 40 minutes

Serves 8

Ingredients:

1 large onion, diced

3 cloves garlic, minced

2 teaspoons

1 tsp cinnamon 2 tsp coriander Zest of 1 orange

2 large sweet potatoes, peeled and chopped 4 cups cooked black beans

3 cups vegetable stock

1 (28-ounce / 794-g) can dice tomatoes, Sea salt, and black pepper to taste

1 cup chopped fresh cilantro (garnish)

2 jalapeño peppers, seeded and finely chopped (garnish)
2 fresh limes, quartered (garnish)

Directions:

1.   Sauté the onion in a large saucepan over medium-high heat for 6 mins. Add the garlic, cumin, cinnamon, coriander, and orange zest. Sauté for 1 minute. Add the sweet potatoes, black beans, and vegetable stock. Bring to a boil, decrease heat, and simmer for 15 minutes until the sweet potatoes are tender. Add the tomatoes and more stock if needed, and cook for another 10 minutes. Add salt and pepper.

2.   Serve garnished with the chopped cilantro and jalapeño peppers, with lime wedges on the side.

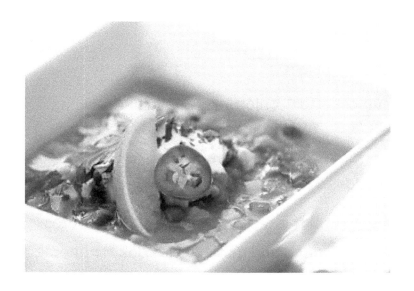

Smoky Black Bean Bisque

Preparation time: 10 minutes

Cook time: 30 minutes

Serves 4

Ingredients:

1 onion 2 cloves garlic

2 tsp cumin seeds 2 tsp oregano

3 chipotle peppers 4 cups black beans

2½ to 3 cups vegetable stock

Sea salt, to taste

1 lime

1 cup cilantro 1 onion

Directions:

1.   Sauté the yellow onion for 8 minutes. Add the cumin, oregano and garlic, then cook for another minute. Add the black beans, vegetable stock and chipotles, then

bring to a boil over high heat. Cook the soup for 20 minutes. Add salt and purée the soup in a blender.

2.   Serve garnished with lime wedges, cilantro, and red onion.

Potato Leek Soup

Preparation Time: 5 Minutes

Cooking Time: 5 Minutes

Servings: 4

Ingredients:

1 cup cilantro leaves 6 garlic cloves, peeled

3 tbsp vegetable oil

3 leeks, white and green parts chopped

2 lb. russet potatoes, peeled and chopped 1 tsp cumin powder

¼ tsp salt

¼ tsp black pepper 2 bay leaves

6 cups no-sodium vegetable broth

Directions:

1.   In a spice blender, process the cilantro and garlic until smooth paste forms.

2.   Sauté the garlic mixture and leeks until the leeks are tender, 5 minutes.

3.   Mix in the remaining ingredients and allow boiling until the potatoes soften 15 minutes.

4.   Turn the heat off, open the lid, remove and discard the bay leaves.

5.   Puree the soup until smooth.

6.   Dish the food and serve warm.

Nutrition: Calories   215   Fat   0   g   Protein   10   g Carbohydrates 20.0 g

Kale White Bean Soup

Preparation Time: 10 Minutes

Cooking Time: 45 Minutes

Servings: 4

Ingredients:

1 Onion, medium & finely sliced 3 cups Kale, coarsely chopped

2 tsp. Olive Oil

15 oz. White Beans

5 cups Vegetable Broth 4 Garlic Cloves

Sea Salt & Pepper, as needed

2 tsp. Rosemary, fresh & chopped 1 lb. White Potatoes, cubed

Directions:

1.   Begin by taking a large saucepan and heat it over medium-high heat.

2.   Once the pan becomes hot, spoon in the oil.

3.   Next, stir in the onion and sauté for 8 to 9 minutes or until the onions are cooked and lightly browned.

4.   Then, add the garlic and rosemary to the pan.

5.   Sauté for a further minute or until aromatic.

6.   Now, pour in the broth along with the potatoes, black pepper, and salt. Mix well.

7.   Bring it to a boil.

8.   Allow it to simmer for 32 to 35 minutes or until the potatoes are cooked and tender.

9.   After that, mash the potatoes slightly by using the back of the spoon.

10.   Finally, add the kale and beans to the soup and cook for 8 minutes or until the kale is wilted.

11.   Check the seasoning. Add more salt and pepper if needed.

12.   Serve hot.

Nutrition: Calories: 198 Fat: 11 Fiber: 1 Carbs: 12 Protein: 12

Black Bean Mushroom Soup

Preparation Time: 10 Minutes

Cooking Time: 40 Minutes

Servings: 2

Ingredients:

2 tbsp. Olive Oil

1 clove of Garlic, peeled & minced

½ cup Vegetable Stock 1 tsp. Thyme, dried

15 oz. Black Beans 1 2/3 cup Water, hot oz. Mushrooms

1 Onion, finely chopped 4 Sourdough Bread Slices Vegan Butter, to serve

Directions:

1.   To begin with, spoon the oil into a medium-sized deep saucepan over a medium heat.

2.   Once the oil becomes hot, stir in the onion and garlic.

3.   Sauté for 7 minutes.

4.   Next, spoon in the mushrooms and thyme. Mix well.

5.   Cook for 8 minutes.

6.   Then, pour the water into the mixture along with the stock and beans.

7.   Simmer until the mushroom is soft.

8.   Pour the mixture to a high-speed blender and pulse for 1 to 2 minutes until it is smooth yet grainy.

9.   Serve and enjoy.

Nutrition: Calories: 400 Fat: 32 Fiber: 6 Carbs: 4 Protein: 25

Broccoli Soup

Preparation Time: 5 Minutes

Cooking Time: 15 Minutes

Servings: 2

Ingredients:

3 cup Vegetable Broth 2 Green Chili

2 cups Broccoli Florets 1 tbsp. Chia Seeds

1 cup Spinach

1 tsp. Oil

4 Celery Stalk

1 Potato, medium & cubed 4 Garlic cloves

Salt, as needed

Juice of ½ of 1 Lemon

Directions:

1.   First, heat the oil in a large sauté pan over medium-high heat.

2.   Once the oil becomes hot, add the potatoes to it.

3.   When the potatoes become soft, stir all the remaining ingredients into the pan, excluding the spinach, chia seeds, and lemon.

4.   Add the spinach and chia seed to the pan.

5.   Turn off the heat after cooking for 2 minutes.

6.   Allow the spinach mixture to cool slightly. Blend the mixture for two minutes or until smooth.

7.   Pour the lemon juice over the soup. Stir and serve immediately.

8.   Enjoy.

Nutrition: Calories: 200 Fat: 3 Fiber: 2 Carbs: 5 Protein: 4

Squash Lentil Soup

Preparation Time: 10 Minutes

Cooking Time: 35 Minutes

Servings: 4

Ingredients:

7 cups Vegetable Broth 2 tbsp. Olive Oil

2 tsp, Sage dried

1 Yellow Onion, medium & diced. Salt & Pepper t0 taste

1 Butternut Squash 1 ½ cup Red Lentils

Directions:

1.   Stir the onions in a saucepan with heated oil.

2.   Sauté the onions for 2 to 3 minutes or until softened.

3.   Once cooked, stir in squash and sage while stirring continuously.

4.   Then, spoon in the lentils, salt, and pepper.

5.   Bring the lentil mixture to a boil for about 30 minutes. Lower the heat.

6.   Then, allow the soup to cool down until the lentils are soft.

7.   Finally, transfer the mixture to a high-speed blender and blend for 3 to 4 minutes or until smooth.

8.   Serve hot.

Nutrition: Calories: 200 Fat: 7 Fiber: 4 Carbs: 7 Protein: 5

Mexican Soup

Preparation Time: 10 Minutes

Cooking Time: 45 Minutes

Servings: 6

Ingredients:

2 tbsp. Extra Virgin Olive Oil

8 oz. can of Diced Tomatoes & Chilies 1 Yellow Onion, diced

2 cups Green Lentils

½ tsp. Salt

2 Celery Stalks, diced 8 cups Vegetable Broth

2 Carrots, peeled & diced

2 cups Diced Tomatoes & Juices 3 Garlic cloves, minced

1 Red Bell Pepper, diced 1 tsp. Oregano

1 tbsp. Cumin

¼ tsp. Smoked Paprika

1 Avocado, pitted & diced

Directions:

1.   Heat oil in a large-sized pot over medium heat.

2.   Once the oil becomes hot, stir the onion, bell pepper, carrot, and celery into the pot.

3.   Cook until the veggies are soft.

4.   Then, spoon in garlic, oregano, cumin, and paprika into it and sauté for one minute or until aromatic.

5.   Next, add the tomatoes, salt, chilies, broth, and lentils to the mixture.

6.   Now, bring the tomato-chili mixture to a boil and allow it to simmer for 32 to 40 minutes or until the lentils become soft.

7.   Check the seasoning and add more if needed.

8.   Serve along with avocado and hot sauce.

Nutrition: Calories: 344 Fat: 23 Fiber: 12 Carbs: 3 Protein: 16

Bean and Mushroom Chili

Preparation time: 15 minutes

Cook time: 38 minutes

Serves 6

Ingredients:

1 large onion, peeled and chopped

1 pound (454 g) button mushrooms, chopped 6 cloves garlic, peeled and minced

1 tablespoon ground cumin

4 teaspoons ground fennel

1 tablespoon ancho chile powder

½ teaspoon cayenne pepper

1 tablespoon unsweetened cocoa powder

4 cups beans 1 can diced tomatoes

Salt, to taste (optional)

Directions:

1.   Put the mushrooms and onion in a saucepan and sauté over medium heat for 10 minutes.

2.   Add the garlic, cumin, fennel, chile powder, cayenne pepper, and cocoa powder and cook for 3 minutes.

3.   Add the remaining ingredients and simmer, covered, for 25 minutes. Season with salt, if desired.

4.   Serve immediately.

Nutrition Per Serving:

calories: 436 | fat: 2g | carbs: 97g | protein: 19g | fiber: 23g

Five-Bean Chili

Preparation time: 10 minutes

Cook time: 1 hour

Serves 8

Ingredients:

2 (26- to 28-ounce / 737- to 794-g) cans diced tomatoes

1 (19-ounce / 539-g) can red kidney beans, drained and rinsed

1 (19-ounce / 539-g) can white kidney beans, drained and rinsed 1 (19-ounce / 539-g) can chickpeas, drained and rinsed

1 (19-ounce / 539-g) can black beans, drained and rinsed 1 (19-ounce / 539-g) can pinto beans, drained and rinsed 2½ cups fresh mushrooms, sliced

1 pepper 1 onion

1 cup corn, canned or frozen

1tbsp chili powder

½ teaspoon freshly ground black pepper

½ teaspoon pink Himalayan salt

¼ teaspoon cayenne pepper

¼ teaspoon garlic powder

Directions:

1.   Mix all the ingredients. Cook, occasionally stirring, for 45 to 60 minutes.

2.   Serve with brown rice, quinoa, or fresh avocado. If you have leftovers or do meal prep, store in reusable containers in the refrigerator for up to 5 days or freeze for up to 2 months.

Nutrition Per Serving:

calories: 756 | fat: 5g | carbs: 139g | protein: 41g | fiber: 44g

Caribbean Bean Chili

Preparation time: 15 minutes

Cook time: 1 hour

Serves 4

Ingredients:

2 tablespoons coconut oil 1 onion, diced

1 green pepper, diced

3 Roma tomatoes, chopped 2 carrots, diced

5 ounces (142 g) tomato paste

2 tablespoons chili powder 1 teaspoon salt

1 teaspoon ground cumin

½ teaspoon cinnamon

½ teaspoon allspice

½ teaspoon dried oregano

½ teaspoon cayenne pepper

¼ teaspoon garlic powder

¼ teaspoon garlic, minced

¼ teaspoon ground black pepper

1 can beans 1 ear corn, kernels cut from the cob

Directions:

1.   Sauté until the onion is translucent, about 10 to 15 minutes.

2.   Add the water, carrots, tomato past and tomatoes. Boil and simmer for 30 minutes.

3.   Mix the beans and the corn, the simmer for another 15 minutes.

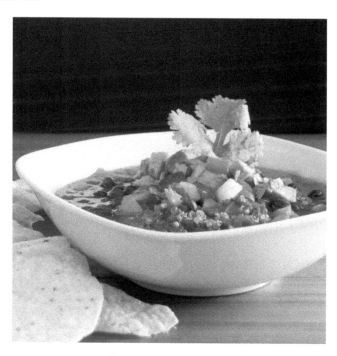

Black Bean Chili

Preparation time: 40 minutes

Cook time: 45 minutes

Serves 8 to 10

Ingredients:

1 medium eggplant, cut into ½-inch cubes 1 cup low-sodium vegetable broth or water 4 cloves garlic, minced

3 onions 1 yellow bell pepper, diced 1 red bell pepper, diced

2 zucchini, chopped

1 (28-ounce / 794-g) can Italian plum tomatoes, with juice 4 large ripe plum tomatoes, diced

½ cup slivered fresh basil leaves

½ cup parsley 2 tbsp chili powder

2 tsp oregano 1 tbsp cumin

1 tsp black pepper

¼ teaspoon crushed red pepper flakes 2 cups cooked black beans

1½ cups frozen corn kernels, thawed

¼ cup fresh lemon juice

½ cup chopped fresh dill

Directions:

1.   Preheat the broiler to High.

2.   Remove and let it cool.

3.   Add the garlic, onions, peppers, and zucchini to the broth, then cook for 10 minutes, stirring occasionally.

4.   On your cutting board, coarsely chop the canned tomatoes and add them to the soup pot, along with their juice. Stir in the fresh tomatoes, basil, parsley, chili powder, oregano, cumin, black pepper, and red pepper flakes. Add the broiled eggplant and simmer covered over low heat for 20 minutes or until the tomatoes are tender.

5.   Add the beans, corn kernels, lemon juice, dill, and mix well. Cook for 10 minutes more.

6.   Allow to cool for 5 minutes and serve warm.

Nutrition Per Serving:

calories: 127 | fat: 1g | carbs: 23g | protein: 5g | fiber: 7g

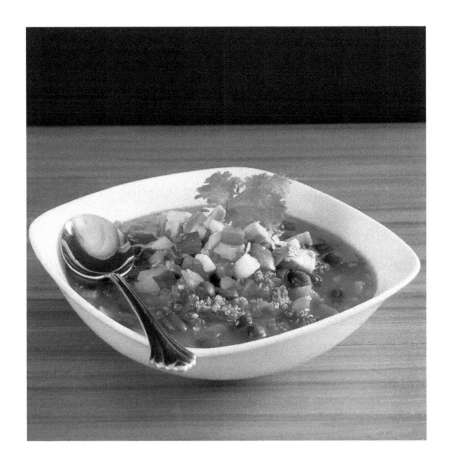

Kidney Bean and Lentil Chili

Preparation time: 20 minutes

Cook time: 51 minutes

Serves 6 to 8

Ingredients:

2 medium bell peppers, deseeded and chopped (about 1 cup) 1½ cups chopped celery

3 carrots (about 1 cup)

3 medium yellow onions, peeled and chopped (about 1½ cups) 1 to 2 cloves garlic, peeled and minced

6 cups low-sodium vegetable broth, divided

1½ tablespoons chili powder

½ teaspoon chipotle powder 1 teaspoon ground cumin

1 teaspoon paprika

½ teaspoon cayenne pepper

1 (15-ounce / 425-g) can beans 2 cups red lentils

1 (28-ounce / 794-g) can crushed tomatoes

Zest and juice of 1 lime

Salt

Directions:

1.   Put the bell peppers, celery, carrots, onion, garlic, and 1 cup of the vegetable broth in a large pot over medium-high heat. Cook, occasionally stirring, until the vegetables soften, 6 minutes.

2.   Add the chili powder, chipotle powder, cumin, paprika, and cayenne pepper and cook for an additional minute, stirring well.

3.   Add the kidney beans, lentils, tomatoes, and the remaining vegetable broth to the pot. Let it boil.

4.   Reduce the heat to medium-low and simmer, occasionally stirring, until the lentils are soft, about 45 minutes.

5.   Season with salt and pepper. Serve immediately.

Nutrition Per Serving:

calories: 352 | fat: 3g | carbs: 63g | protein: 20g | fiber: 14g

Vegetable Broth Sans Sodium

Preparation Time: 5 minutes

Cooking Time: 60 minutes

Servings: 1 cup

Ingredients:

5 sprigs of dill

2 freshly sliced yellow onions 4 chives

6 freshly peeled and sliced carrots 10 cups of water

4 freshly sliced celery stalks

3 cloves of freshly minced garlic 4 sprigs of parsley

Directions:

1.   Put a large pot on medium heat and stir the onions. Fry them until fragrant. Add the garlic, celery, carrots, and dill along with the chives and parsley, and cook everything. You will know that the mix is ready when it becomes fragrant.

2.   Add the water and allow the mixture to boil. Reduce the heat and allow everything to cook for 45 minutes.

3.   Turn off the heat. The broth will cool in about 15 minutes.

4.   Strain the broth with the help of a sieve to have a clear vegetable broth.

Nutrition:

Calories: 362 Carbs: 12g Protein: 12g Fat: 12g

Amazing Chickpea and Noodle Soup

Preparation Time: 10 minutes

Cooking Time: 20 minutes

Servings: 1 cup

Ingredients:

1 freshly diced celery stalk

¼ cup of 'chicken' seasoning 1 cup of freshly diced onion

3 cloves of freshly crushed garlic 2 cups of cooked chickpeas

4 cups of vegetable broth Freshly chopped cilantro

2 freshly cubed medium-size potatoes Salt

2 freshly sliced carrots

½ teaspoon of dried thyme Pepper

2 cups of water

6 oz. of gluten-free spaghetti 'Chicken' seasoning

2 tsp of sea salt

1 1/3 cup of nutritional yeast

3 tbsp of onion powder 1 tsp of oregano

½ teaspoon of turmeric

1 ½ tablespoon of dried basil

Directions:

1.	Put a pot on medium heat and sauté the onion. It will soften within 3 minutes.

2.	Add celery, potato, and carrots and sauté for another 3 minutes

3.	Add the 'chicken' seasoning to the garlic, thyme, water, and vegetable broth.

4.	Simmer the mix on medium-high heat. Cook the veggies for about 20 minutes until they soften.

5.	Add the cooked pasta and chickpeas.

6.	Add salt and pepper to taste.

7.	Put the fresh cilantro on top and enjoy the fresh soup!

Nutrition:

Calories: 405 Carbs: 21g Protein: 19g Fat: 18g

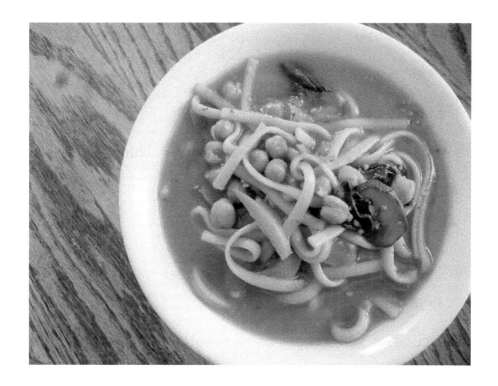

Lentil Soup the Vegan Way

Preparation Time: 5 minutes

Cooking Time: 20 minutes

Servings: 1 cup

Ingredients:

2 tablespoons of water

4 stalks of thinly sliced celery

2 cloves of freshly minced garlic 4 thinly sliced large carrots

Sea salt

2 freshly diced small shallots

 Pepper

3 cups of red/yellow baby potatoes 2 cups of chopped sturdy greens

4 cups of vegetable broth

1 cup of lentils

Fresh rosemary/thyme

Directions:

1.   Put a large pot over. Put in the shallots, garlic, celery, and carrots to water. Season.

2.   Sauté the veggies for 5 minutes until they are tender. You will know that the veggies are ready when they have turned golden brown.

3.   Add the potatoes and some more seasoning. Cook for 2 minutes.

4.   Mix the vegetable broth with the rosemary. Now Increase the heat to medium-high. Allow the veggies to be on a rolling simmer. Add the lentils and give everything a thorough stir.

5.   Once it starts to simmer again, decrease the heat and simmer for about 20 minutes without a cover. You will know that the veggies are ready when both the lentils and potatoes are soft

6.   Add the greens. Cook for 4 minutes until they wilt. You can adjust the flavor with seasonings.

7.   Enjoy this with rice or flatbread. The leftovers are equally tasty, so store them well to enjoy on a day when you are not in the mood to cook.

Nutrition:

Calories: 284 Carbs: 21g Protein: 11g Fat: 19g

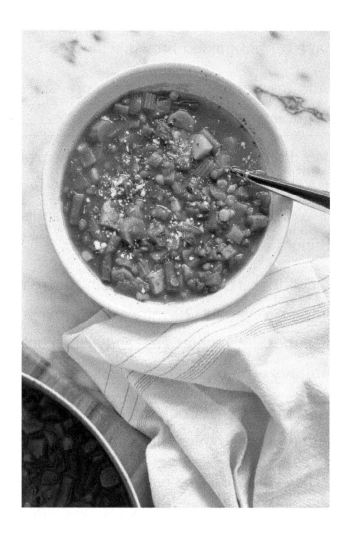

Beet and Kale Salad

Preparation Time: 5 minutes

Cooking Time: 5 minutes

Servings: 1

Ingredients:

8 oz. of beet and kale blend 1 tablespoon of olive oil

1 cucumber

6 oz. of chickpeas Salt

2 tablespoons of red wine vinegar Pepper

¼ cup of walnuts

2 oz. of dried cranberries Cashew cheese

Directions:

1.   Cut the veggies and combine everything in a big salad bowl.

2.   Serve the fresh salad and enjoy a hearty meal.

Nutrition:

Calories: 490 Carbs: 31g Protein: 19g Fat: 21g

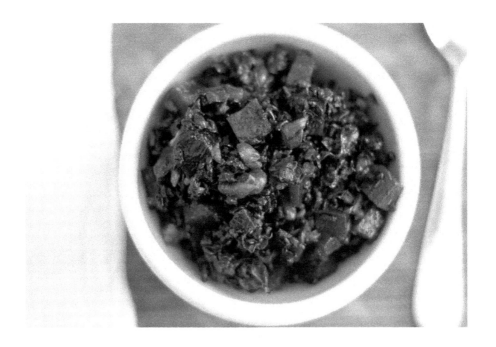

Kale and Cauliflower Salad

Preparation Time: 10 minutes

Cooking Time: 15 minutes

Servings: 1 portion

Ingredients:

6 oz. of Lacinato kale

8 oz. of cauliflower florets 1 lemon

1 tablespoon of Italian spice 2 radishes

oz. of butter beans Olive oil

¼ cup of walnuts

¼ cup of vegan Caesar dressing Pepper

Salt

Directions:

1.   Preheat the oven to 400°F. Toss the cauliflowers with olive oil and spices, and add salt. Roast the cauliflower until it is brown. It will be done within 15-20 minutes.

2.   De-stem the kale and slice the leaves. Slice the radishes. Both kale and radish should be sliced thinly. Cut the lemon in half.

3.   In a large bowl add the the kale and the lemon juice and salt along with the pepper. Massage the kale so that it is appropriately covered with seasoning. The leaves will soon turn dark green. Mix the radishes.

4.   Rinse the butter beans and pat them dry with a towel. On medium-high heat, put a large skillet, add some olive oil, and sauté the butter beans in a layer. Sprinkle some salt on top and shake the pan. The butter beans will be brown in places within 7 minutes.

5.   Take two large plates and divide both the kale and beans equally. Put the walnuts and roasted cauliflower on top. Add the Caesar dressing on top and enjoy the fantastic salad.

Nutrition:

Calories: 378 Carbs: 11g Protein: 18g Fat: 27g

Asian Delight with Crunchy Dressing

Preparation Time: 20 minutes

Cooking Time: 10 minutes

Servings: 1 bowl

Ingredients:

Salad Dressing:

½ teaspoon of powdered ginger or 1 teaspoon of freshly chopped ginger

1 tablespoon of honey

¼ cup of rice wine vinegar 2 tablespoons of soy sauce 3 tablespoons of sesame oil

3 tablespoons of creamy peanut butter

Salad:

¼ cup of vegetable oil

2 tablespoons of toasted sesame seeds

1 finely shredded carrot

1 thinly sliced red bell pepper

6 cups of washed and dried spinach

¼ red onion 1 cucumber

½ pound of snap peas

½ cup of roasted peanuts

1 tablespoon of toasted sesame seeds

Directions:

1.   Whisk the ingredients well. Do not put the sesame seeds in this dressing mixture.

2.   Bring it to a boil. Put the sugar snaps in, then cook until they are crisp and tender. Drain and rinse them repeatedly in cold water so that the peas retain their crispy nature.

3.   Put all the other ingredients in the salad. Put the salad dressing on top so that the veggies are well-coated. Add the toasted sesame seeds. Enjoy this salad when you are not in the mood for anything heavy.

Nutrition:

Calories: 378 Carbs: 11g Protein: 18g Fat: 27g

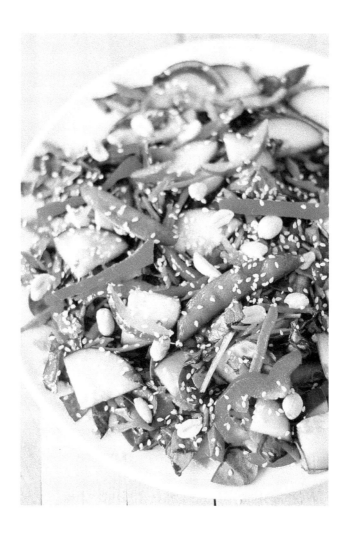

Classic Mixed Bean Chili

Preparation time: 10 minutes

Cook time: 1 hour 30 minutes

Serves 6

Ingredients:

1 pound (454 g) beans, mixed varieties (you can buy premixed or mix your own)

1 tablespoon extra-virgin olive oil

½ cup diced onion

4 cloves garlic, finely chopped

4 cups vegetable broth, more if needed

1 (28-ounce / 794-g) can crushed fire-roasted tomatoes
1 (8-ounce / 227-g) can tomato sauce

1 (6-ounce / 170-g) can tomato paste

2 tbsp Worcestershire sauce 2 tbsp chili

3 tsp ground cumin 1½ teaspoons dried oregano

¼ teaspoon ground cloves

½ teaspoon cayenne pepper 1 teaspoon salt

Directions:

1.   Place the beans in a stockpot. Cover with water by about 3 inches. The beans will swell. Let soak overnight.

2.   Place the beans into the stockpot.

3.   In the heated oil, add the onion and sauté until translucent, about 10 to 15 minutes. Add the garlic and sauté another minute. Place in the stockpot. Add the vegetable broth, crushed tomatoes, tomato sauce, tomato paste, and Worcestershire sauce. A couple of inches of liquid should cover the beans. You can add more broth or water if needed. Stir well. Cover and bring to a boil.

4.   Simmer. Make sure your heat isn't too high. Cook for 1 hour and check the beans. You will want them tender.

Kidney bean and Tomato Chili

Preparation time: 10 minutes

Cook time: 10 to 20 minutes

Makes 4 bowls

Ingredients:

2 to 3 garlic cloves, minced

1 onion, diced

1 to 2 tablespoons water, vegetable broth, or red wine

¼ cup tomato paste or crushed tomatoes 1 (28-ounce / 794-g) can tomatoes

2 to 3 teaspoons chili powder

1 (14-ounce / 397-g) can kidney beans, rinsed and drained, or 1½ cups cooked

¼ teaspoon sea salt (optional)

¼ cup fresh cilantro or parsley leaves

Directions:

1.   Add the garlic, onion, and water in a large pot and sauté for about 5 minutes until the vegetables are softened. Mix in the tomato paste, tomatoes, chili powder, and beans. Sprinkle with salt, if desired.

2.   Bring the mixture to a simmer for at least 10 minutes or until cooked to your preferred doneness, stirring occasionally.

3.   Divide the chili among bowls and serve garnished with cilantro.

Nutrition Per Serving (1 bowl):

calories: 179 | fat: 12g | carbs: 8g | protein: 8g | fiber: 7g

Navy Bean Chili

Preparation time: 15 minutes

Cook time: 35 minutes

Serves 6

Ingredients:

1 large green pepper, deseeded and diced 1 large yellow onion, peeled and diced

3 jalapeño peppers, deseeded and minced 6 cloves garlic, peeled and minced

2 tablespoons ground cumin seeds, toasted

4 cups cooked beans 1 (28-ounce / 794-g) can diced tomatoes

3 cups low-sodium vegetable broth

Zest and juice of 2 limes 1 cup finely chopped cilantro Salt, to taste (optional)

Directions:

1.   Put the green pepper, onion, and jalapeño peppers in a large saucepan and sauté over medium cook for 8 minutes.

2.   Cook for 2 minutes. Add the beans, tomatoes, and vegetable broth and bring to a boil over high heat.

3.   Cook for 25 minutes. Add the lime zest and juice and cilantro and season with salt, if desired.

4.   Serve immediately.

Nutrition Per Serving:

calories: 373 | fat: 8g | carbs: 61g | protein: 15g | fiber: 20g

Lentil Chili

Preparation time: 15 minutes

Cook time: 30 to 35 minutes

Serves 6 to 8

Ingredients:

1 pound (454 g) lentils

8 cups water or low-sodium vegetable broth, plus more as needed 2 cups diced onion

1 cup crushed tomatoes

¼ cup tomato paste

2 tablespoons chopped garlic

2 tbsp vinegar 2 tbsp flime juice 1 tbsp ground cumin

2 tablespoons chili powder

1 teaspoon cayenne (use less if you don't like your chili spicy)

Directions:

1.   Put all the ingredients together and boil over high heat.

2.   Reduce the heat to medium-low and let simmer covered for 30 to 35 minutes, or until the lentils are softened, adding more water or broth if needed for desired chili consistency.

3.   Remove from the heat and serve.

Nutrition Per Serving:

calories: 145 | fat: 1g | carbs: 26g | protein: 7g | fiber: 3g

White Bean Soup with Green Herb Dumplings

Cook time: 25 minutes

Servings: 6

Ingredients

White Bean Soup:

1 can (14 oz.) cannellini beans, drained, rinsed

½ cup whole wheat pastry flour 2 carrots, peeled and diced

3 tablespoons olive oil 5 cups of water

1 big onion, finely chopped 1 teaspoon salt

Green Herb Dumplings:

1 cup herbs (scallions, dill, basil), chopped 2 tablespoons pesto

1 ½ cups whole wheat pastry flour 2 teaspoons baking powder

1 ¼ cup milk

½ teaspoon salt

Directions:

1.   Heat olive oil, then fry onions and carrots in it for about 7 mins. Add flour and cook for 4 minutes. Add water and salt and boil for 6 minutes. Stir in beans and boil while you prepare the herbs.

2.   Mix milk and pesto properly in a bowl, then add herbs.

3.   Put together baking powder, salt and flour. Add the milk mixture, then mix properly to combine. Add a large tablespoon of this mixture into the boiling soup.

4.   Cover and cook for 7 minutes. Flip each dumpling, then cook for extra 7 minutes. Top with more herbs and serve hot.

Celery Dill Soup

Preparation Time: 10 Minutes

Cooking Time: 20 Minutes

Servings: 4

Ingredients:

1 tbsp coconut oil

½ lb. celery root, trimmed 1 garlic clove

1 medium white onion

¼ cup fresh dill, roughly chopped 1 tsp cumin powder

¼ tsp nutmeg powder

1 small head cauliflower, cut into florets 3½ cups seasoned vegetable stock

5 oz. vegan butter Juice from 1 lemon

¼ cup coconut cream

Salt and black pepper to taste

Directions:

1.   Sauté the celery root, garlic, and onion until softened and fragrant, 5 minutes.

2.   Stir in the dill, cumin, and nutmeg, and stir-fry for 1 minute. Mix in the cauliflower and vegetable stock. Bring it to boil.

3.   Add the vegan butter and lemon juice, and puree the soup using an immersion blender.

4.   Stir in the coconut cream, salt, black pepper, and dish the soup.

5.   Serve warm.

Nutrition: Calories: 180 Fat: 12 Fiber: 4 Carbs: 5 Protein: 17

Medley of Mushroom Soup

Preparation Time: 10 Minutes

Cooking Time: 20 Minutes

Servings: 4

Ingredients:

4 oz. unsalted vegan butter

1 onion 1 garlic clove

2 cups sliced mixed mushrooms

½ lb. celery root, chopped

½ tsp dried rosemary 3 cups of water

1 vegan stock cube, crushed 1 tbsp plain vinegar

1 cup coconut cream

6 leaves basil, chopped

Directions:

1.   Sauté the onion, garlic, mushrooms, celery, and rosemary until the vegetables soften 5 minutes.

2.   Stir in the water, stock cube, and vinegar. Cover the pot, allow boiling, and then simmer for 10 minutes.

3.   Mix in the coconut cream and puree the ingredients using an immersion blender until smooth. Simmer for 2 minutes.

4.   Dish the soup and serve warm.

Nutrition: Calories: 140 Fat: 3 Fiber: 2 Carbs: 1. 5 Protein: 7

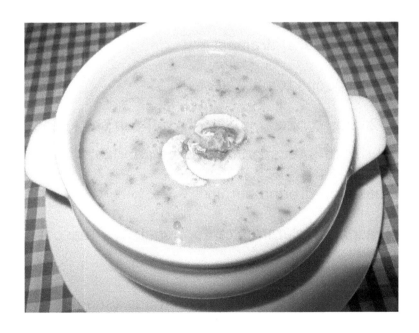

Moroccan Vermicelli Vegetable Soup

Preparation Time: 5 minutes

Cooking Time: 35 minutes

Servings: 4 to 6

Ingredients:

2 tbsp extra-virgin olive oil

2 onions

2 carrots, chopped 1 celery rib, chopped

3 small zucchinis, cut into 1/4-inch dice 1 (28-oz.) can diced tomatoes, drained

2 tablespoons tomato paste

11/2 cups cooked or 1 (15.5-oz.) can chickpeas, drained and rinsed 2 teaspoons smoked paprika

1 teaspoon ground cumin

1 teaspoon za'atar spice (optional) 1/4 teaspoon ground cayenne

6 cups vegetable broth, homemade (see light vegetable broth) or store-bought, or water

Salt

4 oz. vermicelli

2 tablespoons minced fresh cilantro for garnish

Directions:

1.   Add the onion, carrot, and celery in a saucepan. Cook for 6 minutes. Stir in the zucchini, tomatoes, tomato paste, chickpeas, paprika, cumin, za'atar, and cayenne.

2.   Add the broth and salt. Simmer the vegetables until tender.

3.   Shortly before serving, stir in the vermicelli and cook until the noodles are tender about 5 minutes. Garnish and serve.

Nutrition:

Calories: 236 Fat: 1.8g Carbs: 48.3g Protein: 7g

20-Minute Tofu Soup
Preparation time: 40 minutes

Yield: 3 to 4 servings

Ingredients

1 tablespoon (15 ml) neutral-flavored oil

1 teaspoon toasted sesame oil ¼ cup (53 g) minced shallot

¼ cup (40 g) minced garlic

2 teaspoons grated fresh ginger root

8 ounces (227 g) extra-firm tofu, drained, pressed, cut into skinny slices, then into ½-inch (6 mm) pieces

½ cup plus 2 tablespoons (90 g) daikon matchsticks

3 tablespoons (43 g) minced carrot ½ teaspoon ground white pepper

½ tsp pepper 2½ cups (590 ml) vegetable broth

3 tablespoons (45 ml) tamari

1 tablespoons (30 ml) seasoned rice vinegar

1 teaspoon to taste Minced scallion for garnish

Directions:

1.   Heat the oils in a medium-size saucepan over medium heat. Add the shallot, garlic, and ginger. Cook for 3 minutes, occasionally stirring, until fragrant.

2.   Add the tofu, daikon, carrot, white pepper, and cayenne pepper. Some of the tofu may break, and that is okay. Cook for 2 minutes, stirring.

3.   Add the broth, tamari vinegar, and sambal oelek.. Cook for 10 minutes serves garnished with scallion.

Vegan Cauliflower Soup

Cook time: 25 minutes

Servings: 6 Ingredients

Ingredients:

1 head (3-pound) cauliflower, cut into florets 2 cups split peas, cooked

2 tablespoons dietary yeast 2 tablespoons olive oil

7 cups of water

1½ yellow onions, chopped   1 ½ teaspoon ground turmeric Black pepper, to taste

1 ½ teaspoon salt

Instructions:

1.   Add onions, turmeric, and salt in heated olive oil and cook for about 10 minutes, stirring infrequently.

2.   Bring it to a boil. Add cauliflower and cook for 20 minutes. Add yeast and remaining water, then let it boil uncovered for about 5 minutes.

3. Blend the soup with a blender until smooth. Add more water and salt if necessary, then add the black pepper and serve with split peas.

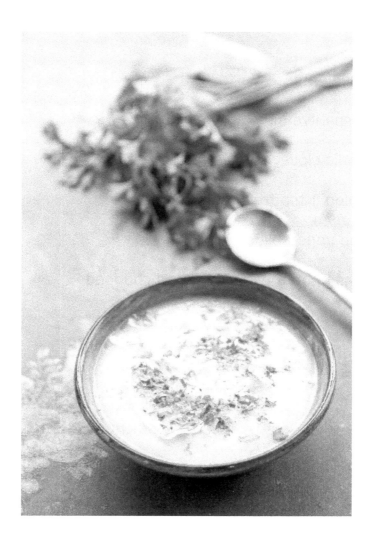

Tofu and Mushroom Soup

Preparation Time: 15 Minutes

Cooking Time: 10 Minutes

Servings: 4

Ingredients:

2 tbsp olive oil

1 garlic clove, minced

1 onion 1 tsp freshly grated ginger

1 cup vegetable stock

2 small potatoes, peeled and chopped

¼ tsp salt

¼ tsp black pepper

2 (14 oz) silken tofu, drained and rinsed 2/3 cup baby Bella mushrooms, sliced 1 tbsp chopped fresh oregano

2 tbsp chopped fresh parsley to garnish

Directions:

1. Sauté the garlic, onion, and ginger until soft and fragrant.

2. Pour in the vegetable stock, potatoes, salt, and black pepper. Cook until the potatoes soften, 12 minutes.

3. Stir in the tofu, and using an immersion blender, puree the ingredients until smooth.

4. Mix in the mushrooms and simmer with the pot covered until the mushrooms warm up while occasionally stirring to ensure that the tofu doesn't curdle, 7 minutes.

5. Stir oregano, and dish the soup.

6. Garnish with the parsley and serve warm.

Nutrition: Calories 310 Fat 10 g Protein 40.0 g Carbohydrates 0 g

Avocado Green Soup

Preparation Time: 5 Minutes

Cooking Time: 5 Minutes

Servings: 4

Ingredients:

2 tbsp olive oil

1 ½ cup fresh kale, chopped coarsely

1 ½ cup fresh spinach, chopped coarsely

3 large avocados, halved, pitted, and pulp extracted 2 cups of soy milk

2 cups no-sodium vegetable broth 3 tbsp chopped fresh mint leaves

¼ tsp salt

¼ tsp black pepper 2 limes, juiced

Directions:

1.   Mix in the kale and spinach in heated olive oil. Cook until wilted, 3 minutes, and turn off the heat.

2.   Puree the soup until smooth.

3.   Dish the soup and serve immediately.

Nutrition:

Calories 400 Fat 10 g Protein 20 g Carbohydrates 30 g

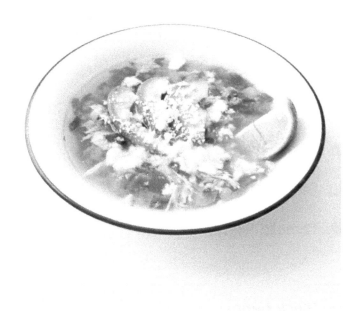

Black Bean Nacho Soup

Preparation Time: 7

Minutes Cooking Time: 35 Minutes

Servings: 4

Ingredients:

30 oz. Black Bean 1 tbsp. Olive Oil

2   cups Vegetable Stock

½ of 1 Onion, large & chopped 2 ½ cups Water

3   Garlic cloves, minced

14 oz. Mild Green Chillies, diced 1 tsp. Cumin

1 cup Salsa

½ tsp. Salt

16 oz. Tomato Paste

½ tsp. Black Pepper

Directions:

1.   For making this delicious fare, heat oil in a large pot over medium-high heat.

2.   Once the oil becomes hot, stir in onion and garlic to it.

3.   Sauté for 4 minutes or until the onion is softened.

4.   Next, spoon in chili powder, salt, cumin, and pepper to the pot. Mix well.

5.   Then, stir in tomato paste, salsa, water, green chilies, and vegetable stock to onion mixture. Combine.

6.   Bing the mixture to a boil. Allow the veggies to simmer.

7.   When the mixture starts simmering, add the beans.

8.   Bring the veggie mixture to a simmer again and lower the heat to low.

9.   Finally, cook for 15 to 20 minutes and check for seasoning. Add more salt and pepper if needed.

10.   Garnish with the topping of your choice. Serve it hot.

Nutrition: Calories 270 Fat 10 g Protein 10 g
Carbohydrates 10 g

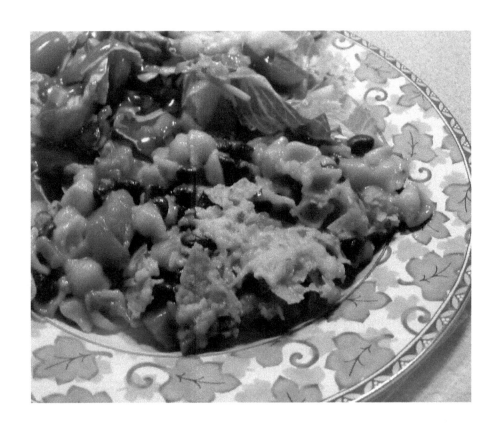

Thyme Watercress and Potato Soup

Preparation time: 10 minutes

Cook time: 40 minutes

Serves 4 to 6

Ingredients:

2 large leeks, diced

3 cloves garlic, minced

1 teaspoon minced fresh thyme

5 potatoes 5 cups vegetable stock

2 bunches of watercress, chopped

Sea salt and pepper, to taste

Directions:

1.   Sauté the leeks in a large saucepan over medium heat until softened. Cook for 2 minutes adding salt and thyme. Put in the potatoes and vegetable stock, then bring to a boil. Cover the pot, decrease the heat to medium, and cook until the potatoes are tender about 20

mins. Add the watercress and cook for 5 mins. Purée in a blender and return to a pan over low heat.

2.   Season and finish cooking.

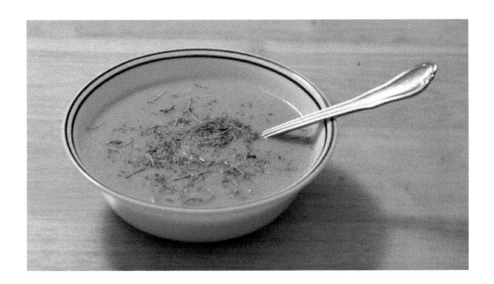

Southwestern Potato Corn Chowder

Preparation time: 15 minutes

Cook time: 30 minutes

Serves 6

Ingredients:

1 large yellow onion, diced into ¼-inch cubes 1 large red bell pepper, diced into ¼-inch cubes

4 ears corn (about 3 cups) 3 cloves garlic

2 tsp cumin seeds 2 jalapeño peppers, minced

½ cup finely chopped fresh cilantro 6 cups vegetable stock

2 large potatoes, cut into ¼-inch pieces Sea salt and black pepper, to taste

Directions:

1. Sauté the onion and red bell pepper over medium heat for 7 to 8 minutes. Add the corn, garlic, cumin, jalapeño peppers, cilantro, and cook for 2 minutes. Add the vegetable stock and potatoes, and bring the pot to a

boil. Cook for 15 minutes or so until the potatoes are tender.

2.   Cook for a few minutes more adding salt and pepper.

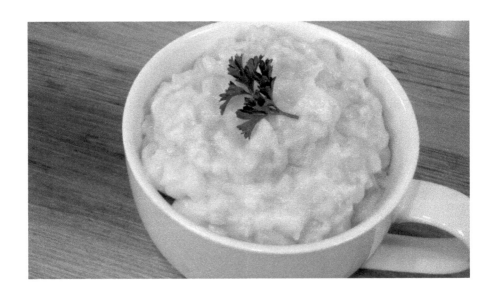

Vegetable Curry Noodle Soup

Preparation time: 10 minutes

Cook time: 35 minutes

Serves 4

Ingredients:

½ onion, chopped

3 garlic cloves, minced

1-inch fresh ginger root, peeled and minced 4 cups vegetable broth, divided

2 cups unsweetened plant-based milk

½ block firm tofu, cubed 1 cup snap peas

1 cup bean sprouts

1 cup chopped mushrooms 1 tablespoon curry paste

1 teaspoon curry powder 1 teaspoon turmeric

1 teaspoon freshly ground black pepper 2 ounces (57 g) wide rice noodles

Directions:

1.   Sauté the onion, garlic, and ginger in ¼ cup of broth until softened. Add the milk, the rest of the broth, tofu, snap peas, bean sprouts, mushrooms, curry paste, curry powder, turmeric, and pepper. Leti t cook for 25 to 30 minutes, stirring occasionally. Add the noodles, stir, cover, and cook for another 5 minutes, or until the noodles are soft.

2.   Serve and enjoy!

Nutrition Per Serving:

calories: 161 | fat: 4g | carbs: 24g | protein: 9g | fiber: 5g

The Mediterranean Delight with Fresh Vinaigrette

Preparation Time: 5 minutes

Cooking Time: 10 minutes

Servings: 2

Ingredients:

Herbed citrus vinaigrette:

3 tbsp of lemon (juiced) 3 tbsp of orange (juiced)

½ teaspoon of lemon zest

½ teaspoon of orange zest 2 tablespoons of olive oil

1 tablespoon of finely chopped fresh oregano leaves Salt to taste

Black pepper to taste

2-3 tablespoons of freshly julienned mint leave Salad:

1 freshly diced medium-sized cucumber 2 cups of cooked and rinsed chickpeas

½ cup of freshly diced red onion

2 freshly diced medium-sized tomatoes 1 freshly diced red bell pepper

¼ cup of green olives

½ cup of pomegranates

Directions:

1.   Put together the juice and zest of both the lemon and the orange and oregano and olive oil. Whisk together so that they are mixed well. Season the vinaigrette with salt and pepper to taste.

2.   After draining the chickpeas, add them to the dressing. Then, add the onions. Give them a thorough mix so that the onion and chickpeas absorb the flavors.

3.   Now, chop the rest of the veggies and start adding them to the salad bowl. Give them a good toss.

4.   Lastly, add the olives and fresh mint. Adjust the salt and pepper as required.

5.   Serve this Mediterranean delight chilled — a cool summer salad that is good for the tummy and the soul.

Nutrition:

Calories: 286 Carbs: 29g Protein: 1g Fat: 11g

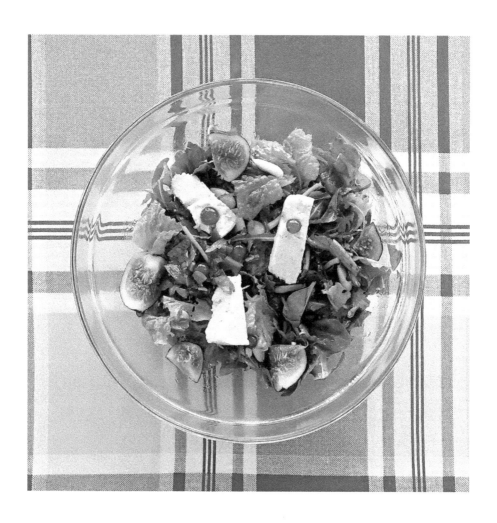

Broccoli Salad the Thai Way

Preparation Time: 10 minutes

Cooking Time: 25 minutes

Servings: 1 portion

Ingredients:

1 tablespoon of tamari

¾ cup of mung beans 1 lime

2 garlic cloves

3 tablespoons of cashew butter 1 cucumber

¼ oz. of fresh mint

1 tablespoon of chili-garlic sauce 1 head of artisan lettuce

3 Thai chilis

6 oz. of broccoli florets

2 tablespoons of olive oil Salt

Pepper

Directions:

1.   On high heat, add the mung beans to 3 cups of cold water. After they start boiling, reduce the heat to medium. Allow the beans to simmer, but stir them from time to time. The mung beans will be tender within 20 minutes. Drain the excess water and add some salt.

2.   Mince the garlic and cut the lime in half. Put together the lime juice, minced garlic, tamari, and cashew butter with chili- garlic sauce. Add 3 tablespoons of warm water. Whisk the mixture well.

3.   Slice the cucumber, cut the broccoli into bite-size pieces, and chop the lettuce. Pick the mint leaves as well. Lastly, slice the Thai chilis.

4.   On a non-stick skillet, put 2 tablespoons of olive oil. Turn the heat to medium-high. Add broccoli. Cook until they are brown. They will be crisp-tender. Add some pepper and salt to the broccoli, and add the lime juice and Thai chilis.

5.   In a shallow bowl, spread some cashew sauce. Add some chopped lettuce, mung beans, broccoli, and cucumber. Add mint leaves and mix the Thai chilies. Add some more cashew sauce, and enjoy the salad!

Nutrition:

Calories: 203 Fat: 1.4g Carbs: 41.6g Proteins: 4.8g

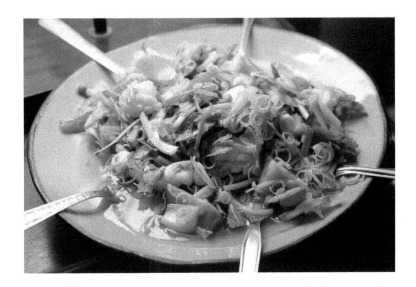

Sweet Potato, Corn and Jalapeno Bisque

Preparation Time: 10 minutes

Cooking Time: 15 minutes

Servings: 4

Ingredients:

4 ears corn

1 seeded and chopped jalapeno 4 cups vegetable broth

1 tablespoon olive oil

3 peeled and cubed sweet potatoes 1 chopped onion

½ tablespoon salt

¼ teaspoon black pepper 1 minced garlic clove

Directions:

1.   In a pan, heat the oil over medium flame and sauté onion and garlic in it, and cook for around 3 minutes. Put broth and sweet potatoes in it and bring it to boil. Reduce the flame and cook it for an additional 10 minutes.

2.   Blend with a blender. Again, put it on the stove and add corn, jalapeno, salt, and black pepper and serve it.

Nutrition:

Calories 332 Carbs: 31g Protein: 6g Fat: 4g

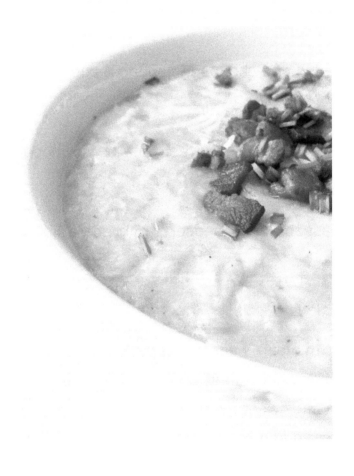

Creamy Pea Soup with Olive Pesto

Preparation Time: 20 minutes

Cooking Time: 20 minutes

Servings: 4

Ingredients:

1 grated carrot

1 rinsed chopped leek 1 minced garlic clove 2 tablespoons olive oil

1 stem fresh thyme leaves

15 oz. rinsed and drained peas

½ tablespoon salt

¼ tsp black pepper 2 ½ cups vegetable broth

¼ cup parsley leaves

1 ¼ cups pitted green olives 1 teaspoon drained capers

1 garlic clove

Directions:

1.   Take a pan with oil and put it over medium flame, and whisk garlic, leek, thyme, and carrot in it. Cook it for around 4 minutes.

2.   Add broth, peas, salt, and pepper, and increase the heat. When it starts boiling, lower down the heat and cook it with a lid on for around 15 minutes and remove from the heat and blend it.

3.   For making pesto, whisk parsley, olives, capers, and garlic and blend it so that it has little chunks. Top the soup with a scoop of olive pesto.

Nutrition:

Calories: 230 Carbs: 23g Protein: 6g Fat: 15g

Spinach Soup with Dill and Basil

Preparation Time: 10 minutes

Cooking Time: 25 minutes

Servings: 8

Ingredients:

1 pound peeled and diced potatoes 1 tablespoon minced garlic

1 teaspoon dry mustard 6 cups vegetable broth

20 oz. chopped frozen spinach 2 cups chopped onion

1 ½ tablespoons salt

½ cup minced dill 1 cup basil

½ teaspoon ground black pepper

Directions:

1.   Whisk onion, garlic, potatoes, broth, mustard, and salt in a pan and cook it over the medium flame when it

starts boiling, low down the heat, and covers it with the lid and cook 20 minutes.

2.   Add the remaining ingredients in it and blend it and cook it for few more minutes and serve it.

Nutrition:

Calories: 165 Carbs: 12g Protein: 13g Fat: 1g

Lightning Source UK Ltd.
Milton Keynes UK
UKHW021850300421
382942UK00003B/208